AF228946

Medical Careers in the Military

Gail Snyder

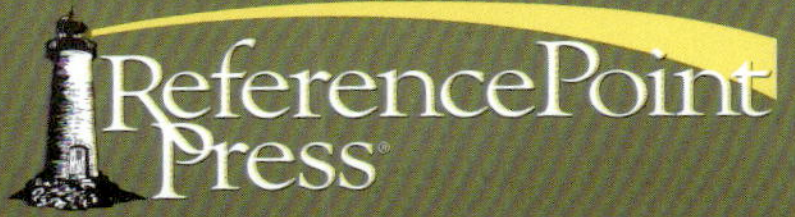

ReferencePoint Press®

San Diego, CA

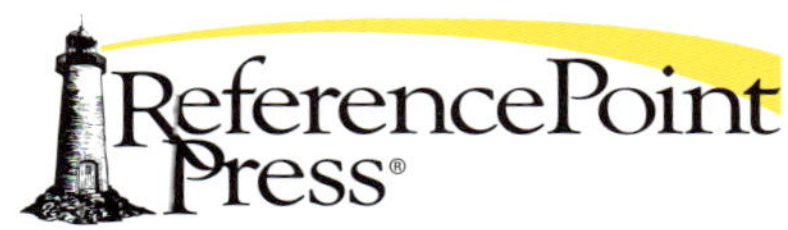

For more information, contact:
ReferencePoint Press, Inc.
PO Box 27779
San Diego, CA 92198
www.ReferencePointPress.com

LIBRARY OF CONGRESS CATALOGING-IN-PUBLICATION DATA

Names: Snyder, Gail, author.
Title: Medical careers in the military / by Gail Snyder.
Description: San Diego, CA : ReferencePoint Press, 2023. | Series: Careers
  in the military | Includes bibliographical references and index.
Identifiers: LCCN 2021056484 (print) | LCCN 2021056485 (ebook) | ISBN
  9781678202941 (library binding) | ISBN 9781678202958 (ebook)
Subjects: LCSH: Medicine, Military--Study and teaching.
Classification: LCC RC971 .S625 2023 (print) | LCC RC971 (ebook) | DDC
  616.9/8023--dc23/eng/20211122
LC record available at https://lccn.loc.gov/2021056484
LC ebook record available at https://lccn.loc.gov/2021056485

Contents

Introduction: An Essential Role

When considering career options, working for one of the world's largest employers—the US military—deserves consideration. This is especially true for young people thinking about a career in health care. After all, as of March 2020 the military was providing free or subsidized health care for 2.1 million active-duty service members and their dependents as well as 19 million more veterans. To do so, it must have enough dentists, physicians, laboratory technicians, nurses, optometrists, occupational therapists, medics, surgeons, psychologists, and more.

According to the Bureau of Labor Statistics' *Occupational Outlook Handbook*, as of 2021 some 65,777 enlisted people were employed in health care jobs by the US Army, Navy, and Air Force, and another 25,865 were officers. Officers—among them lieutenants, captains, and majors—are the managers of the military world. Enlisted people—among them sergeants, corporals, and privates—carry out their orders. Another option is to serve as a part-time member of the military's health care team in the Army, Navy, or Air Force Reserves. Reservists may be called into active duty during an emergency, but in the meantime, they receive military training, job training, a salary, and health care benefits. There are two branches of the military that do not have their own medical personnel. The Marine Corps' medical needs are met by Navy health professionals, and the Coast Guard relies on the US Public Health Service to meet its needs. The Coast Guard is an agency of the Department of Homeland Security.

Serving the Troops and the Nation

Whether performed by someone who is enlisted, an officer, or a reservist, armed forces health care jobs can be found on military bases in clinics, hospitals, and laboratories as well as aboard ships, submarines, helicopters, and airplanes. Such jobs provide an opportunity to serve the troops and the country at the same time—to play a part in the readiness of America's military personnel around the world.

General Sharon Bannister, who is the chief of the Air Force Dental Corps, describes joining the military as a dentist in words that resonate not just with dentistry and the Air Force but also with other health care jobs in the armed forces:

> Military dentistry affords the opportunity to practice with other professionals of all dental and medical specialties to ensure the optimal health of a very special population. It also is a great way to compete for dental school scholarships and potentially secure specialty training to support a low [or] no-cost education. Most importantly, as an Air Force officer, you are part of something much larger than dentistry—you are integral to the success of the mission ensuring the freedoms and safety of the United States of America. . . . I've been able to deploy to areas where I've been able to impact the health of another nation making our world as a whole a healthier place. . . . It is something bigger that has become an integral part of who I am. Put simply, it's not a job; it's truly a way of life. You don't work for the Air Force, you are in the Air Force.[1]

Indeed, there are perks to being in the military. Such benefits may include job training, housing allowances, a salary while in school, signing bonuses, and travel. Also, the military may provide financial assistance to college students who have taken out thousands of dollars in loans to pay for their educations.

Not for Everyone

Still, the military is not for everyone. Applicants have to be at least seventeen years old, US citizens, have normal color vision, and

Sample Military Pay Scales, 2022

Basic pay for military personnel, whether enlisted or officers, is based on years of service and rank. The person's rank usually corresponds with his or her pay grade. Individuals with more years of service and higher rank achieve higher pay grades. As in the civilian world, basic pay is subject to taxes. Some military personnel supplement their income with allowances for housing, clothing, and other needs. Special and incentive pays, such as for hardship duty, can also increase income.

A Sample of Monthly Active-Duty Enlisted Pay Scale for 2022 (all branches)

Years of Service

Sample Pay Grades	<2	2	3	4	6	8	10
E-2	$2,054.72	$2,054.72	$2,054.72	$2,054.72	$2,054.72	$2,054.72	$2,054.72
E-3	$2,160.71	$2,296.58	$2,435.84	$2,435.84	$2,435.84	$2,435.84	$2,435.84
E-4	$2,393.32	$2,515.94	$2,652.12	$2,786.76	$2,905.38	$2,905.38	$2,905.38
E-5	$2,610.22	$2,786.15	$2,920.79	$3,058.51	$3,273.25	$3,497.55	$3,682.10
E-6	$2,849.31	$3,135.53	$3,274.18	$3,408.51	$3,548.70	$3,864.19	$3,987.74
E-7	$3,294.21	$3,595.53	$3,733.56	$3,915.33	$4,057.99	$4,302.62	$4,440.65

A Sample of Monthly Active-Duty Officer Pay Scale for 2022 (all branches)

Years of Service

Sample Pay Grades	<2	2	3	4	6	8	10
O-1	$3,477.22	$3,619.56	$4,375.64	$4,375.64	$4,375.64	$4,375.64	$4,375.64
O-2	$4,006.53	$4,562.65	$5,254.95	$5,432.73	$5,544.26	$5,544.26	$5,544.26
O-3	$4,636.60	$5,255.88	$5,672.43	$6,185.42	$6,482.12	$6,807.16	$7,017.29
O-4	$5,273.75	$6,104.39	$6,512.31	$6,602.58	$6,980.62	$7,386.39	$7,891.67
O-5	$6,112.09	$6,885.42	$7,361.74	$7,451.40	$7,749.33	$7,926.80	$8,318.08
O-6	$7,331.86	$8,054.66	$8,583.36	$8,583.36	$8,616.32	$8,985.43	$9,034.42

E = Enlisted   **O** = Officer

Source: Brittany Crocker, "2022 Military Pay Charts," The Military Wallet, December 29, 2021. https://themilitarywallet.com.

pass fitness tests. They will undergo some version of basic training to learn military culture and must be comfortable following orders. They may need to take tests to determine whether they are suitable for the jobs they seek. In fact, they may end up in different jobs than they expected because that is where the military has the greatest need.

Moreover, when recruits enter the military, they must sign a contract specifying the length of service they will be required to provide. Those who enlist do so for two to four years. Those who enter the military as officers—such as those who are studying to be doctors, physical therapists, and dentists—are required to provide one year of service for every year of financial support they receive from the military during their studies. This can range from five to ten years or even longer. And there is no guarantee that those years will be spent in cities or even countries that candidates would prefer.

For those who opt to make the military their career, they can expect to receive promotions in rank, salary, and job duties. And when it comes time to leave the service, the civilian world will likely welcome their health care skills, leadership experience, and the service they provided their country.

Physician

What Does a Physician Do?

Whether they specialize in skin care, the way the brain works, sleep disorders, or how bodies work in aircraft or space, or whether they read X-rays and ultrasounds or are generalists caring for adults and children, doctors focus on providing the best possible health care to the populations they serve. Students may enlist in the US Army, Navy, or Air Force when they are accepted to medical school or are still in medical school. Or, they may enlist in the first few years after leaving medical school during a time in the careers of young doctors when they are known as "residents." They may also enlist as full-fledged practicing physicians. After joining the service, their duties would be similar to those practiced by civilian doctors: they examine patients, decide what tests to run, interpret the results of those tests, prescribe drugs when necessary, and monitor the effectiveness of the treatment plans they set in motion. What they do is less unusual than where they may be doing it, perhaps in a hospital for veterans, aboard ships or aircraft, or at clinics for soldiers, sailors, aviators, and their families. They may also perform

A Few Facts

Minimum Educational Requirements
Doctor of medicine or doctor of osteopathy degree

Personal Qualities
Analytical, communicative, dexterous, detail oriented, empathetic

Working Conditions
Clinics, hospitals, ships, submarines, airplanes, tents

Salary
Varies by rank and length of service

Future Job Outlook
Need for doctors expected to continue

their duties while deployed in foreign countries and even near battlefields.

Many aspiring physicians join the military for its considerable benefits, which accrue while they serve their country. Such was the case for Colonel Shahid Zaidi, who joined the Air Force in part because the military paid for his tuition to medical school. But he also discovered much more in the bargain. "When I initially joined the Air Force it was about a scholarship and a way to feel like I was giving something back to my country. Now, after almost 19 years, it has been an incredible opportunity," says the physician who serves at Keesler Air Force Base in Mississippi. "Air Force medicine has brought me experiences I wouldn't have had as a civilian. It has allowed me to serve one of the best populations around, our military members and their families."[2]

A Typical Workday

With so many types of physicians in the military, there is no typical day that will cover all specialties. Still, insight into how doctors spend their time in the military can be obtained by examining the days of several physicians: a flight surgeon in the Air Force, a Navy doctor who specializes in treating cancer, and an Army physician who treats everyday ills.

As a flight surgeon, Hernando J. Ortega Jr. performs physical examinations of pilots to ensure that they are able to endure the rigorous demands of flying jets that are capable of traveling hundreds of miles per hour—circumstances that can place physical stresses on their bodies. He also treats ill patients in the base clinic. During his career, he has been asked to serve on a team that investigates accidents involving aircraft, has taken part in emergency response exercises, and has conducted safety briefings and training sessions for astronauts who are expected to perform space walks. He has also flown in military aircraft, serving as the onboard medical officer.

Navy oncologist Jonathan Forsberg treats cancer patients at Walter Reed National Medical Center in Bethesda, Maryland. One of his recent patients was a man whose cancer required the removal of part of his shinbone. Forsberg restored the bone's functionality by surgically implanting a steel plate and screws in the patient's shin. His duties have also included medical research. One task he has been assigned is to help design better-fitting prosthetics—artificial arms and legs—for soldiers who lose limbs in combat.

Army physician Mimi Raleigh's typical day begins at 7:30 a.m. and ends at 4:30 p.m. During those hours, she is likely to see twenty patients or more at the Army's family medicine clinic at Fort Leavenworth, Kansas. She says, "It's a family medicine clinic, so we take care of everything. We perform well-child exams. . . . We do procedures like knee injections, shoulder injections, and biopsies. You almost never know what's going to be coming through the door."[3]

Education and Training

Anyone who wants to be a physician must first complete four years of medical or osteopathy school (a type of medicine that emphasizes bone and muscle conditions), followed by a three- to seven-year residency that takes a deeper dive into their areas of specialization. But before they can do any of that, they must first complete their bachelor's degree with a high grade point average: at least a 3.6 out of 4, meaning they must attain at least a high B average. Then they will need to do well on the Medical Comprehensive Admission Test, which measures their knowledge of biology and physical sciences.

Future doctors who want to serve in the military can begin doing so as soon as they are accepted by an accredited medical school. Signing up early allows medical school students to have their tuition paid for by the military instead of taking out loans that average more than $250,000. They can also receive money for living expenses as well as salaries while they complete their studies.

Medical students who aspire to military careers can opt to attend civilian medical schools or attend the military's own medical school, Uniformed Services University of the Health Services

The First Army Doctor in Space

Military doctors can be found in many places. As the first Army doctor in space, Lieutenant Commander Andrew Morgan proved that some unique frontiers can be traversed by combining the military and medicine. An emergency room physician, Morgan was a crew member on Expedition 60/61, which docked with the International Space Station in 2019. Before he got his seat aboard the Russian rocket that catapulted him into space, he trained for six years, learning everything from how to speak Russian to how to maintain equipment in the space station and walk in space. During his nine months on the space station, his duties included performing scientific experiments.

"At the core, I was selected as an astronaut because they saw a unique set of skills," Morgan says. "Everything I brought to the table was given to me by the Army—my undergraduate and graduate education, residency, and operational experiences." Morgan was also mindful of those who came before him. He carried an armband into space that had been worn by a World War II combat medic.

Quoted in Elaine Sanchez, "NASA Set to Launch First Army Doctor into Space," Military.com, June 14, 2018. www.military.com.

(USUHS) in Bethesda. USUHS students learn the ins and outs of being in the military while they also learn the art of medicine. They wear uniforms to class, and their instructors come from both the civilian and military worlds.

Still, most medical students attend a nonmilitary medical school and have their tuition paid through the military's Health Professions Scholarship Program, to which they must apply. They receive military training by attending modified versions of basic training when it fits into their schedules. Whatever choices they make, medical school students spend the first two years in classrooms and laboratories. During their third year, they begin having some supervised patient contact as they cycle through different specialties to determine what type of medicine they want to practice.

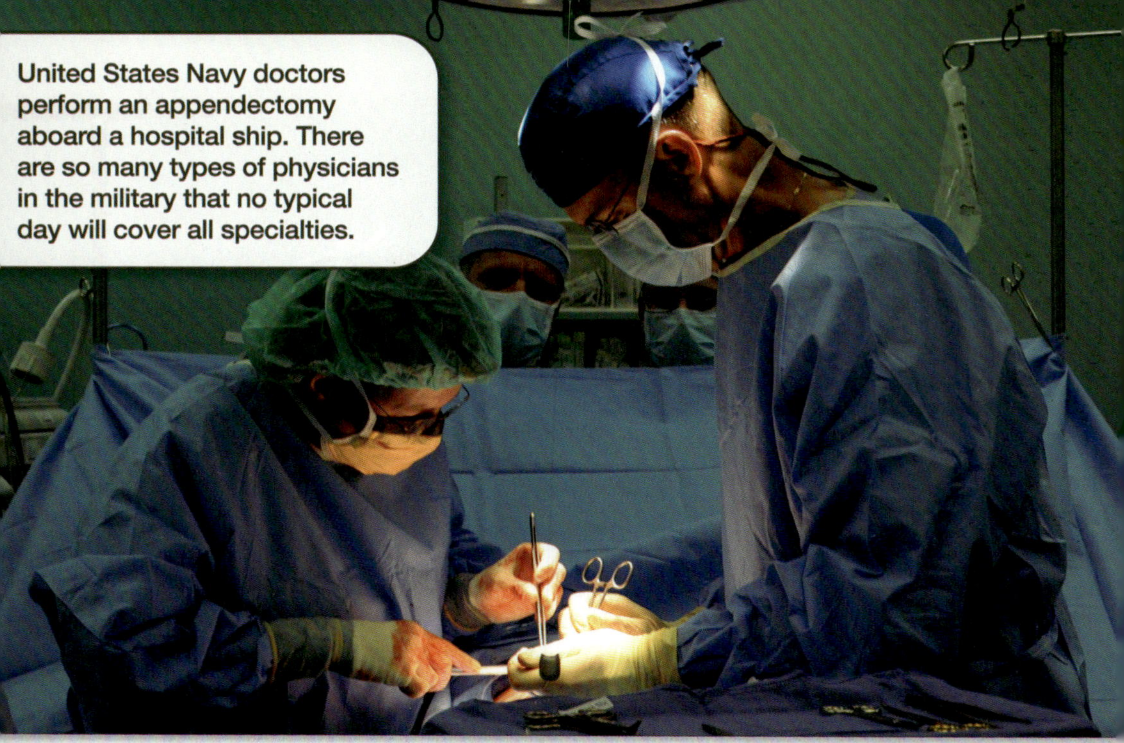

Skills and Personality

Being a physician requires more than intelligence. It requires the ability to communicate so that patients understand what is wrong with them and what they might need to do to get better. The best doctors are also compassionate people who try to be aware of their own biases and look at their patients as people, not just as illnesses. They need to be professionals who smile and have good people skills.

Physicians also have to be willing to share bad news with patients and their families, to answer uncomfortable questions, and to do all they can for patients without doing them harm. They also need to have courage to admit mistakes because, as most experts agree, doctors do sometimes make mistakes. Military physicians may also need to draw on their inner strength when risking their own lives to care for others in war zones or amid disease outbreaks.

Working Conditions

Working conditions will vary depending on whether the doctors are serving on military bases or aboard ships or aircraft. They may be assigned to hospitals in the United States or on foreign bases. Sometimes they find themselves administering care beneath tents near battle zones. Some locations offer state-of-the-art equipment, but others lack the tools and supplies doctors often need. Jesse Shaw practiced medicine aboard submarines, where he often had to make do with medication shortages and limited imaging options despite treating the Navy's elite warriors, its SEALs. (*SEAL* stands for "sea, air, and land." SEALs perform special operations that often require courage and great skills with military weapons, such as breaking into a terrorist lair to free hostages.) Still, Shaw says, "our . . . skills often grow very quickly, because we have to do more with less."[4]

Hanging Out with Pilots

"After graduating from medical school, I was going to become a plastic surgeon. I had no idea about aerospace medicine; never heard of it. I attended medical school on a Health Professions Scholarship Program for the Air Force. During my Air Force surgery internship, I cared for many military retirees who had served in World War II, Korea and Vietnam. Some were pilots and regaled me with stories of their flight surgeons and the unique situations they found themselves in with their flight docs around the world, both in training and in combat. No two stories were alike. They encouraged me to try out being a flight surgeon before 'growing up' in medicine. At the time, anything sounded better than every-other-night [on] call! So, I volunteered to be a flight surgeon and went to an overseas F-16 fighter unit. What a great time: great patients, challenging medicine, world travel, and flying in fighter jets. I haven't looked back."

—Hernando J. Ortega Jr., Air Force flight surgeon

Quoted in American Medical Association, "What It's Like in Aerospace Medicine: Shadowing Dr. Ortega," August 14, 2019. www.ama-assn.org.

Also stressful is when a physician is assigned to work outside his or her specialty. As Kevin Jubbal, a physician who helps guide medical students into careers, explains,

> Military medicine requires a greater level of flexibility and creativity than civilian medicine. Think of the generalist having to perform specialist surgeries while deployed. Additionally, you will have to work in austere, unique, and changing environments. Military medicine can be practiced in active war zones, areas recovering from conflict, pandemics . . . humanitarian missions, global training exercises, and areas subject to natural disasters such as hurricanes.[5]

Opportunities for Advancement

Medical students enter the Army and Air Force as lieutenants. In the Navy, they enter the service in the comparable rank of ensign. Upon graduation, Army and Air Force physicians are promoted to captain, and in the Navy they move up in rank to lieutenant. Military doctors can progress into teaching roles, serve as advisers to their units, be part of research, and participate in humanitarian missions.

They may find themselves like Taylor George, an emergency medicine resident at the Naval Medical Center Portsmouth in Virginia, who says, "I have an exciting field that I have carved for myself, and if I were a civilian provider, I would never have been able to do these things."[6]

Employment Prospects in the Civilian World

When they leave the military, physicians can expect to join an average job market in their field, which is estimated to grow by at least 4 percent through 2029. Substantial growth in the profession is expected as the population ages and develops age-related diseases that need attention. Outside the military, physicians may find jobs in private practice and as part of hospital systems, universities, and pharmaceutical companies.

Pharmacist

What Does a Pharmacist Do?

Most people know pharmacists fill prescriptions written by physicians—in other words, when a doctor orders a prescription drug for a patient, the patient obtains the drug at a local pharmacy. The pharmacist is responsible for providing the drug in the correct quantity and dosage to the patient. Moreover, pharmacists are responsible for determining whether the physician prescribed the correct dosage and for noticing whether the drug may negatively interact with other drugs the patient is taking. But pharmacists also do a lot more.

Pharmacists answer their customers' questions about medicines and share the best way to take them. They may also combine some medicines to fill prescriptions. They are record keepers. They provide vaccinations for flu, COVID-19, and other diseases. Pharmacists also supervise pharmacy technicians who work under them; these techs count out pills required for prescriptions, package and label prescriptions, and organize inventory.

Military pharmacists have additional duties. They provide routine medications for service members with high blood pressure, asthma, and other chronic conditions. They also make sure troops being deployed have sufficient supplies of these

A Few Facts

Minimum Educational Requirements
Doctorate degree

Personal Qualities
Analytical, detail oriented, good communicator

Working Conditions
Hospitals, clinics, tents, ships

Salary
Varies by rank and years of service

Future Job Outlook
More jobs likely with projected wave of retirements

and other medications. They supply pilots with prescription drugs that prevent them from becoming drowsy during long flights and monitor members of the service who have sustained injuries so they do not become addicted to the painkilling drugs they are prescribed.

Moreover—as with any member of the armed services— pharmacists risk being uprooted from their homes, and their own lives may be endangered when they are deployed. Certainly, concerns associated with this unpredictability may add to the stress of being a military pharmacist.

A Typical Workday

Anna Wong currently works as a pharmacist at Benning Martin Army Community Hospital (BMACH), serving in the hospital's outpatient center. (The outpatient center serves patients who have not been admitted to the hospital, meaning they are not staying overnight.) The hospital services Fort Benning in Georgia. In a typical day, she and her colleagues fill as many as four hundred prescriptions during a ten-hour period. She says, "The best part of my job at BMACH is being able to provide focused customer care and service. . . . I enjoy the patient interactions at the BMACH Outpatient Pharmacy."[7]

Wong's daughter Alana is also a military pharmacist assigned to BMACH. But a typical day for Alana is much different than what her mother experiences. Alana serves as a pharmacist for the Fort Benning hospital's medical surgery and intensive care units. Here is how Alana describes her typical day:

> I work closely with the inpatient medicine team to develop optimized care plans for our patients. I work with our inpatient nurses to coordinate the Meds to Beds service, which provides discharge prescriptions and counseling to patients ready to go home. As new medicines and guidelines come out, it's my job to be informed so we can

provide the best care for our patients. This can be challenging as sometimes, like with the [COVID-19] pandemic, the amount of new information coming out can be overwhelming. Each patient has unique factors that should be considered. This is why working with the team is great because we're learning together . . . and can collaborate on a medication regimen that works specifically for this patient at this time.[8]

Life as a Coast Guard Pharmacist

In charge of protecting maritime safety along America's coastlines, the US Coast Guard employs more than thirty-eight thousand members whose health needs must be met. With a vital function but small numbers, the service branch borrows its pharmacists from the US Public Health Service. It relies on just 15 active-duty pharmacists who work at its 150 sites.

As the pharmacy officer for the Coast Guard base in Portsmouth, Virginia, Commander Benjamin C. Keller says that working for such a small enterprise means that he gets to do a lot: the staff includes just Keller and two pharmacy techs. He counsels about twelve service members each day, sometimes advising them on giving up smoking or eating a healthier diet. When service members deploy, he arranges for them to be vaccinated. "We send people all over the world. And a lot of times, they require vaccinations that aren't commercially available within the United States," Keller explains. "So, it creates challenges."

Keller splits his day between clinical work, dispensing drugs, and working with medical personnel—known as corpsmen—aboard the eight Coast Guard vessels he oversees. He is responsible for making sure they have the medications they need to treat patients while also guiding them on the proper dispensing of the prescription drugs.

Quoted in Kate Traynor, "Readiness, Variety Are Hallmarks of Coast Guard Pharmacy," *American Society of Health-System Pharmacists,* January 11, 2017. www.ashp.org.

Education and Training

Becoming a military pharmacist requires a doctorate degree (PharmD) from an accredited pharmacy school. Students can earn an undergraduate degree before applying to pharmacy school, or they can enroll in a six-year program that lets them earn both degrees at once. It is also possible to enlist in the military as a pharmacy technician and then, after gaining experience, progress on to pharmacy school.

As undergraduates, students would do well to take math and science classes to gain foundations in chemistry, physics, and biology. To be accepted into an accredited pharmacy school requires a high grade point average and score on the Pharmacy School Admission Test.

Pharmacy school is expensive, which makes loan repayment programs offered by the military attractive options for many students. In addition, the schooling is rigorous. Students spend time in classrooms studying chemistry, the ways drugs work in human bodies, and ethical issues, such as preserving patient privacy. They also rotate through possible areas of specialization. They must do an internship—professional learning experiences done under close supervision—and, after graduation, pass a licensing examination. Looking back on her first year in pharmacy school, student Erin Mays recalls,

> I never knew I could learn so much in a year. Besides my core pharmacology classes, I had a class on pharmacokinetics, learning how a drug works in the body and how to make dose adjustments based on patient-specific factors, as well as a class on pharmaceutics, learning the ins and outs of the drug development process. Throughout all of these classes, a patient case was always included in every lecture so we were able to see how that information we were learning could be applied to a real-life scenario.[9]

Jacob King is a 2021 PharmD graduate of the University of Colorado's Anschutz Medical Campus in Aurora who planned to enter the Navy after graduation. While at Anschutz, he served a one-year internship at a community pharmacy, where he reveled in his experiences working with customers. He says, "This past year has given me so much experience with patients, and I love the interaction and being able to help someone by explaining what medications they are taking, how the prescriptions metabolize, how it all works together. I think with COVID-19, people are taking more of an active role in their health, and they want to know more about their medications."[10]

After graduation, new pharmacists will spend two years working under the guidance of more experienced pharmacists. Some will add a residency to become a specialist, perhaps in pediatric pharmacy or critical care, where they will learn how to treat patients who are extremely ill. Since military pharmacists are also in the service, they will also need to attend officer training school to learn about the culture of the armed forces.

Skills and Personality

Young people considering careers as pharmacists should ask themselves these questions: Are they detail oriented? Does the idea of learning the uses and possible side effects of scores of medications—and their interactions—appeal to them? Can they picture themselves talking to patients of varying ages and answering their questions about their health conditions? Would they be comfortable telling the people who work for them, the pharmacy techs, what to do? Pharmacists need to be good communicators. They also need to order supplies, manage inventory, and keep records—all of which require attention to detail.

"All pharmacists have to be capable of practicing pharmacy with competence and know where to find the information to take care of the patient," says Captain Rohin Kasudia, the executive officer for the Sixth Medical Group at MacDill Air Force Base in

Ready for Anything

"My role is to make sure service members have safe and effective medications. We have to be ready to open a pharmacy anywhere in the world. My job is to make sure our service members get the same level of pharmaceutical care there that you or I would get in Boston. . . . I enjoy the challenge. I don't just have to know about pain and [end of life] care. I have to understand the logistics of getting meds where they need to go; I have to understand how to make those medications in austere environments; I have to communicate how to use those medications; along with all the other skills that I learned [in pharmacy school]. At the time I attended, we didn't get a whole lot of logistics and supply—but there may be more of that in the curriculum now that medication shortages are a bigger part of the landscape."

—Ryan Costantino, a pharmacist and the director of Pharmacy Clinical Decision Support for the Defense Health Agency

Quoted in Massachusetts College of Pharmacy and Health Sciences University, "'Go Where the Need Is': Major Ryan Costantino Pharmd '12 Shares His Outlook on Pharmacy." www.alumni.mcphs.edu.

Tampa, Florida. "But fundamentally, the Air Force wants pharmacists with leadership and integrity who can inspire and empower those around them. I think it is the characteristics like that which can really distinguish military pharmacists."[11]

Working Conditions

Working conditions will vary depending on whether pharmacists are working in a hospital, aboard a ship, or in the field. Those assigned to hospitals will experience fairly routine days and few medication shortages. Pharmacists on ships or in the field may have to work around medication shortages and fewer amenities.

All military pharmacists face daily pressures. Not only do they need to process prescriptions accurately and quickly, but they also need to make certain troops that are deploying have all the medicines they need for the time period they may be away. Also, like all military personnel, military pharmacists face the uncertainties of being deployed at any time or being called away for training exercises. Burnout can be a problem. As Colonel Hope Williamson-Younce, the director of the Army System for Health Directions, explains, "They can deploy with field hospitals during times of conflict . . . for extended periods of time. The threat of bodily harm in combat environments is also stressful. So not only are they taking care of their patients, but they have to exercise their survivability skills."[12]

Opportunities for Advancement

Pharmacists enter the military as officers and are eligible to rise through the ranks. Pharmacists who do rise in the ranks take on increasingly greater responsibilities. They might become more involved with administrative duties that will eventually take them further away from the day-to-day demands of running pharmacies or even being pharmacists.

Many military pharmacists truly love their jobs and are very happy with their career paths. In a 2015 survey of 276 retired military pharmacists with twenty years or more of service reported by the journal *Military Medicine*, nearly 92 percent said they would take the same career path if they had to do it over again.

Employment Prospects in the Civilian World

If military pharmacists choose to enter the civilian world, they may find the number of jobs is on a slight decline, with seven thousand fewer jobs expected to be filled through 2030 compared to the decade before, according to the Bureau of Labor Statistics' *Occupational Outlook Handbook*. Still, there will always be a need for pharmacists, and jobs will continue to open up as pharmacists retire. Moreover, as Americans grow older as a nation, they are likely to require more medications to keep their chronic conditions at bay. Industry-wide changes, such as the rise of online pharmacies, may lead to a shifting of where pharmacists are employed.

Still, there are expected to be many jobs available for pharmacists in health care settings such as hospitals and clinics, where older patients are expected to make up a good percentage of patients coming in with more illnesses to be treated. As civilian pharmacists, military veterans could work for a big chain, such as CVS or Walgreens, or perhaps own their own neighborhood pharmacies. They might also find employment in hospital pharmacies.

Laboratory Specialist

What Does a Laboratory Specialist Do?

Military laboratory specialists usually work behind closed doors in labs where they conduct tests on tissue samples and blood, urine, and spinal fluids while wearing protective gloves, clothing, and goggles. Often that means examining a specimen under a microscope or growing cell cultures in Petri dishes, which are small, shallow dishes used in biological analyses. Through the efforts of laboratory specialists, physicians are able to identify the sources of illnesses, such as tiny insects and microscopic viruses that live off of human hosts, and determine the appropriate treatment for eliminating them.

Not long ago, Brayden Bex, a laboratory specialist in the Army, found himself leaving the confines of the laboratory for a more public role because of the spread of COVID-19. Stationed in Germany and attached to the Landstuhl Regional Medical Center's Infectious Disease Laboratory, Bex and his fellow lab workers found themselves playing vital roles in attempting to tamp down a pandemic. He did so by processing COVID-19 test samples so that soldiers would know whether they were contagious and in danger of spreading the sometimes fatal virus. The Alexandria, Kentucky, native expressed gratitude for the opportunity to carry out this highly visible duty:

> I have been given the privilege to be part of this COVID virology team [a group that examines viruses] and work through complex testing which is greater than my typical scope of work. This has shown me the impact of my job on the health care system. . . . I contribute to overall Army readiness by performing COVID-19 testing and assisting with data collection for future dissection that could lead to a possible change in how we approach training, transportation, and our daily lives.[13]

Laboratory specialists sometimes collect the specimens as well as test them. For example, they may need to insert a needle to draw blood from a patient's vein and carefully store the sample until it can be tested. Samples need to be kept free of contamination and stored at the right temperature so they can be properly analyzed.

Laboratory specialists can also assist with blood bank work. Blood collected for future use must be tested to identify its type (such as A, B, and O) so that people who need blood transfusions receive the correct type. Lab specialists may also package blood supplies to be shipped to remote locations where they are needed. Lab specialists also need to be familiar with laboratory functions and equipment, including how to set up a lab, dismantle it, and put it back together in a new and perhaps temporary location.

A Typical Workday

A typical workday for a lab technician may start in the lab by donning a lab coat, checking the machines, and then cleaning, repairing, or calibrating them for the tests that need to be performed during that shift. In a single day, these lab workers might perform a variety of tests using different machines. One commonly used machine is a centrifuge, whose spinning action separates liquids. Another is a chemical analyzer, which is set up to automatically conduct tests on samples of blood or other body fluids. A typical day might require the technician to repeatedly conduct a single type of test—for example, testing throat swabs for the presence of COVID-19 or classifying blood types.

At any moment, that work might need to be put aside should a test with emergency priority come in that must be accomplished quickly. With people's lives at stake, all work has to be double-checked by the lab specialist before generating a report to the physicians who authorized the tests.

Education and Training

In order to be a laboratory specialist, enlistees will need either an associate's or a bachelor's degree in medical technology or

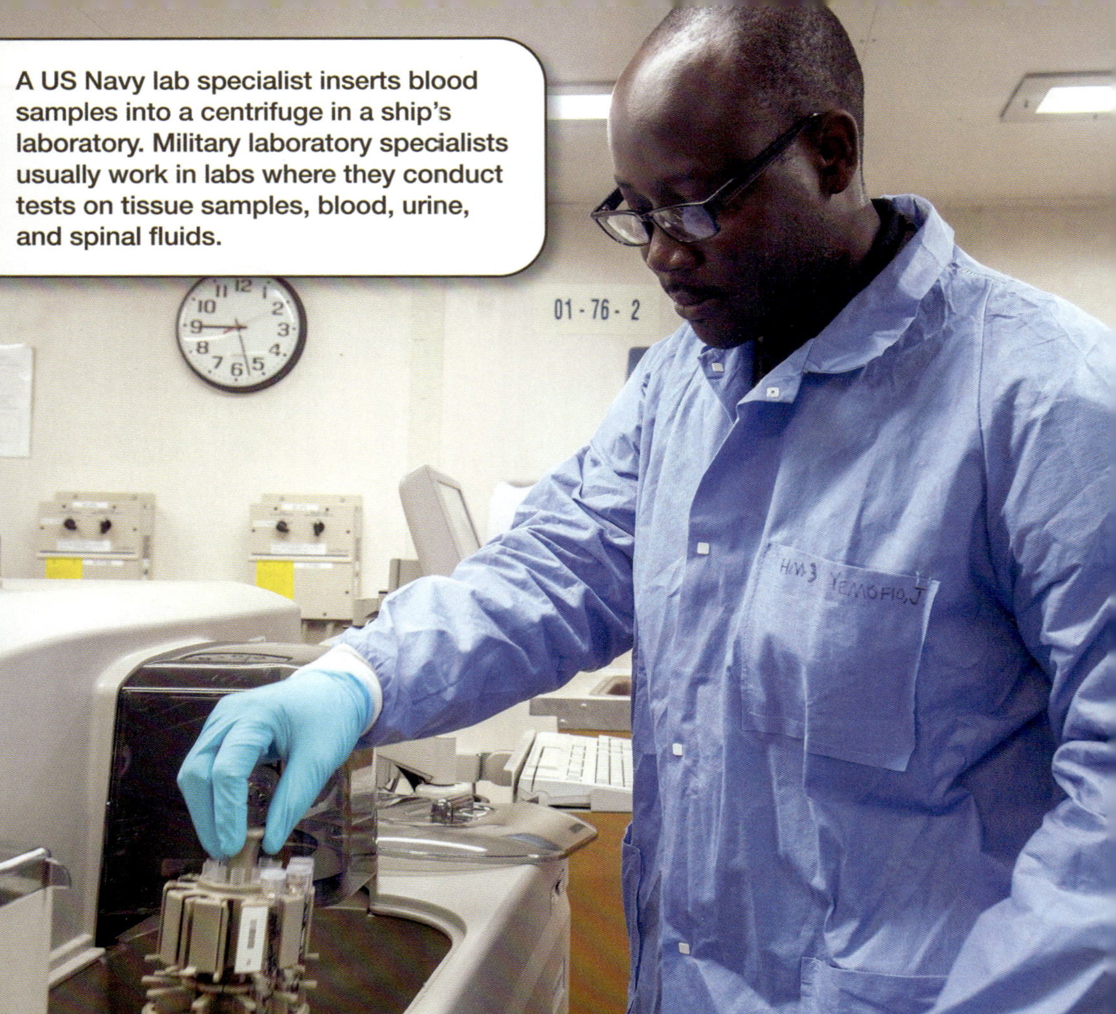

A US Navy lab specialist inserts blood samples into a centrifuge in a ship's laboratory. Military laboratory specialists usually work in labs where they conduct tests on tissue samples, blood, urine, and spinal fluids.

another scientific field of study. They also need a high score on the skilled technical portion of the Armed Services Vocational Aptitude Battery (ASVAB). Developed by the Department of Defense, the ASVAB measures the test taker's strengths to determine where he or she might be best utilized. If the prospective job applicant proves to be a match for the position of laboratory specialist, and there are openings at the time, he or she will first need to complete basic training. During this ten-week period, new recruits learn the skills typically expected of members of the Army, Navy, or Air Force—among them, how to work as a team, how to handle weapons, and how to perform under pressure. What follows next will vary depending on the service branch. In the Army, the service member will spend a year training at a military hospital and, after that, will receive additional instruction on lab procedures, record keeping, and administrative duties.

What separates military laboratory specialists from those who work in civilian jobs is a military culture focusing on discipline. "If I had to cite the major difference between ours and a civilian program, it is the level of discipline required to succeed in the military,"[14] says Major Michael D. Miller, the chief of education and training at the US Army Medical Department Center and School at Fort Sam Houston in San Antonio, Texas. In a typical day, Miller explains, students rise from their beds at 4:30 a.m. and spend a busy day going to classes and studying until lights out at 10 p.m.

Skills and Personality

A laboratory specialist cannot be squeamish when it comes to blood, tumor cells, or microorganisms such as bacteria and viruses. Just as an understanding of biology, chemistry, and algebra is essential to the job, so are good oral and written communication skills. Furthermore, prospective laboratory specialists need to keep their workstations neat and uncluttered, be capable of carrying out detailed procedures, and have above-average hand-eye coordination.

Laboratory specialists spend a good portion of their days on their feet, so they need to have good physical stamina too. It is also important to have a suitable personality for the job: laboratory specialists must be team players who are also able to work independently, dependably, and analytically.

Working Conditions

Laboratory specialists work in military hospitals and laboratories. It may be necessary to work weekends or odd hours during emergency situations or deployments. Laboratories maintain antiseptic environments to avoid spreading germs and diseases and specimen contamination. But that does not mean that the people who work in them are not warm and friendly.

K.C. Geisler, who works in the laboratory department at the naval base in Bremerton, Washington, says the best part of his career has been the closeness he has experienced with his work mates. "It is never about the duty station that you go to. It's all about the relationships that you build with the people you work with that really matters. In the laboratory we are a family. People that join the Navy—or any other service branch for that matter—typically are not in close proximity to their families. So we adopt each other and take care of one another."[15]

Opportunities for Advancement

The longer a person spends in the military, the more likely he or she is to receive promotions in rank, increases in salary, additional education opportunities, and a variety of assignments. Colonel Noel R. Webster's career illustrates that point. Webster's Army career began with training as a laboratory specialist, but he also went on to receive master's degrees in hospital administration and biology. He also earned certification in blood collection. His military career has been marked by continual advancement, rising from laboratory supervisor to medical platoon leader, medical company commander, lab manager, director of a blood donor center, and laboratory program manager. His military duties have, at times, taken him to other countries. According to Webster,

> The most unusual situation was my six-month lab management rotation to Honduras. I tested for some parasitic diseases I would never have seen in the United States. I worked with some Honduran civilian hospital laboratories, and flew to remote sites to help people in need of medical care. It was very educational and enlightening to visit many different countries, working with scientists around the world.[16]

Employment Prospects in the Civilian World

Prospects for laboratory specialists in the civilian world are very good, with the profession expected to grow by 7 percent through 2029, with the addition of about twenty-five thousand new jobs, according to the Bureau of Labor Statistics' *Occupational Outlook Handbook*. The increase in demand for the profession seems assured because of an aging population's tendency to develop more health conditions that will need laboratory tests to diagnose.

As they leave the military, laboratory specialists are likely to find employment in hospitals, where 47 percent of the jobs are expected to be. The next-largest employers of these specialists are private companies that operate commercial laboratories, such as Labcorp and Quest Diagnostics, where 20 percent of the jobs will be found. (Commercial laboratories such as those operated by Labcorp and Quest Diagnostics typically analyze samples taken in physicians' offices, or take samples in their own neighborhood locations.) There will also be a smaller number of jobs in physicians' offices, outpatient care centers, and university research centers. For people who enjoy working in the clean, quiet, and orderly atmosphere of a laboratory and carrying out medical tests that will help resolve patients' medical conditions, working as a civilian laboratory specialist may prove satisfying.

What Does a Registered Nurse Do?

Of all the health care professionals in the military, registered nurses (RNs) spend the most time caring for patients. Their patients may be active members of the military, their family members, or veterans. As members of the Nurse Corps who come on board as officers, RNs employed by the Army, Navy, Air Force, and Coast Guard need a bachelor's degree in nursing. Their duties include chronicling patient medical histories, measuring blood pressure, taking temperatures, giving immunizations, keeping records, dispensing medications authorized by physicians, and screening patients to determine whether they need to be seen by physicians.

If they work in a military hospital, their duties might include wound care, surgical care, infant care, or care for senior citizens. Registered nurses work closely with physicians and are responsible for carrying out the latters' orders, monitoring their patients, and sharing information with physicians.

A Typical Workday

Workdays for RNs vary depending on the type of nursing involved and where that nursing takes place—in the field, in a hospital, or in a clinic. And there is great variety in the possible

---

A Few Facts

Minimum Educational Requirements
Bachelor's degree

Personal Qualities
Caring, detail oriented, communicative

Working Conditions
Hospitals, clinics, ships, tents

Salary
Varies by rank and years of service

Future Job Outlook
Above average: projected growth rate of 19 to 26 percent

specializations. In the Navy, for example, RNs can work in critical care, with patients whose illnesses require constant monitoring to avoid death; neonatal care, with the tiniest newborns who may need help breathing or gaining weight before they can go home; pediatrics, with young children; or surgical units, working with patients before, during, or after surgery. Some Navy RNs also do research.

In addition, as RNs bounce from one assignment to the next, their typical days will change considerably. Lieutenant Colonel Leesa Harrie spent more than five years in the Army Nurse Corps.

Improving the Lives of Burn Patients

RNs interested in wound care and research have made important contributions in the military. Before Army nurse Elizabeth Mann-Salinas retired from the military, she had developed methods for treating soldiers who had sustained burns that left them in terrible pain. During her twenty-three-year military career, Mann-Salinas served as a head nurse, senior nurse scientist, and head of the Joint Trauma System (JTS). The mission of the JTS is to determine the care practices that lead to favorable outcomes in patients who have been injured in battle. The Army paid for her master's degree in clinical nursing and gave her the opportunity to do research in Afghanistan on trauma care and help develop a technique for improving kidney function in burn patients. (When someone receives a severe burn their damaged tissue may lead to poor blood flow to their kidneys, lessening their ability to efficiently rid the body of waste material.)

She became a pioneer in improving burn patients' lives. "I fell in love with their passion to live. . . . They have multiple medical issues that come from the burns and the subsequent inflammatory response, and then they face rehabilitation and the lifelong struggle of living as a burn patient," she explains.

Quoted in Diane Szulecki, ed., "Pioneering Military Burn Research," *American Journal of Nursing*, September 2019, vol. 119, no. 9. www.nursingcenter.com.

After nursing school, the Army assigned her to work with cancer patients for a few years. She then worked at Walter Reed National Medical Center in Bethesda, Maryland. There, she was assigned to a section of the hospital where both officers and enlisted men and women were treated for a variety of conditions.

Education and Training

Registered nurses must have a bachelor's degree in nursing and accreditation through the National Council Licensure Examination. The pass/fail computerized exam, which is given by the National Council of State Boards of Nursing, evaluates whether recent nursing students know enough to begin practicing.

Although the military hires nurses who have completed their education and have two years of work experience, it also offers scholarship opportunities for students who are in nursing school to help pay for their education. Although there are accelerated nursing school programs, most programs take four years to complete. The curriculum combines classroom study with clinical experience.

In addition to receiving training in nursing, military RNs need to become acclimated to life in the armed forces. They learn what they need to know by enrolling in a commissioned officer course. Captain Lisa Dukes of the Army Nurse Corps describes the course this way:

> Medical personnel in the Army take a basic officer leader course. . . . But, no one is yelling in our face or forcing us to do push-ups (although I guess they could). The course is 11 weeks long. The first two weeks are introductory. . . . We also get three weeks of field training where we sleep in a tent, carry a weapon, and do simulated convoy exercises. It's nothing like what enlisted soldiers go through—it's a much lighter version. The Army recognizes that nurses are already professionals. For the most part, this training course is the easiest time I have spent in the military.[17]

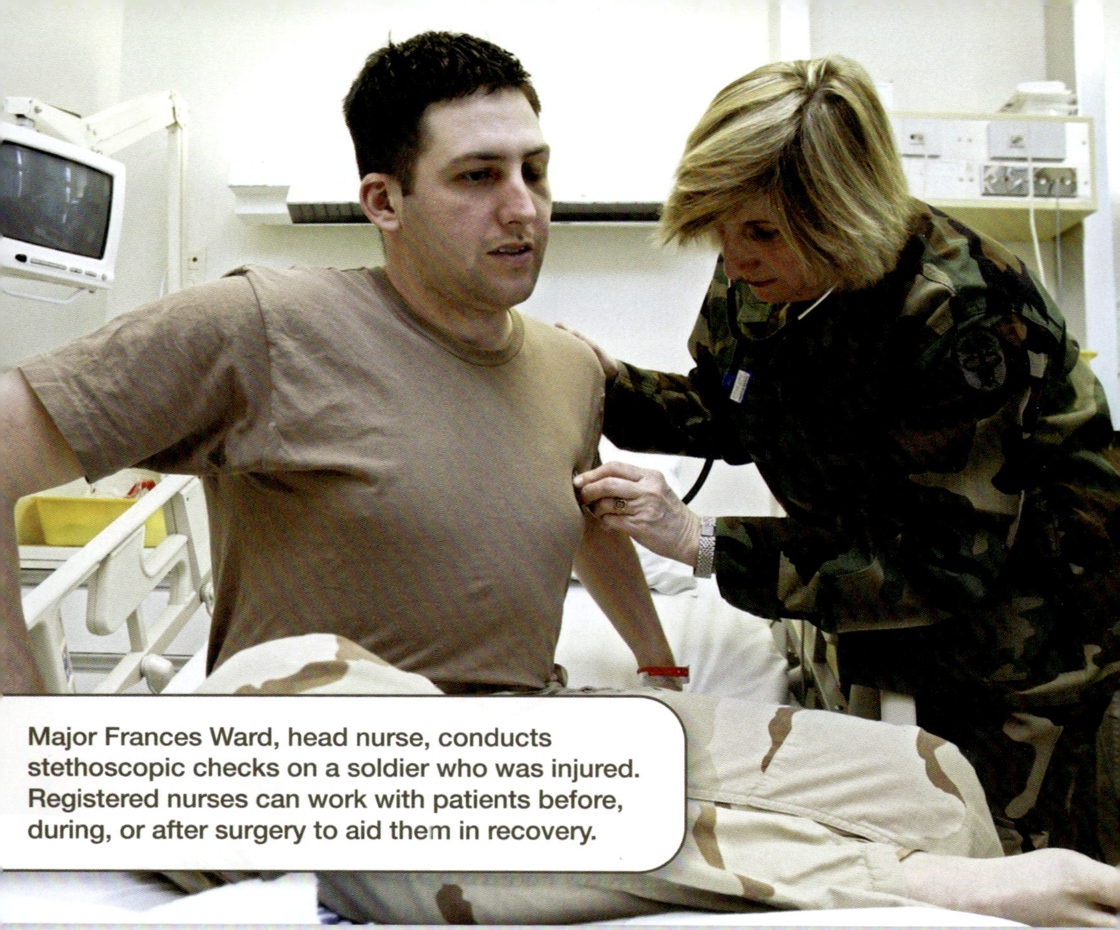

Major Frances Ward, head nurse, conducts stethoscopic checks on a soldier who was injured. Registered nurses can work with patients before, during, or after surgery to aid them in recovery.

Skills and Personality

To be effective, RNs require many attributes, not the least of which is compassion for the sick, injured, and those in pain. Nurses need to be calm and authoritative but good listeners too. They need to communicate important information about illness and self-care to patients because they are the ones who work directly with them. They act as intermediaries in carrying out doctors' orders. As military officers, they need to demonstrate leadership and good decision-making and organizational skills. They also need to speak up when they see something amiss that needs correcting. For example, RNs may need to tell their supervisor if they suspect a physician has prescribed the wrong dosage or a dangerous medication or if a patient is not responding as anticipated to a treatment.

Working Conditions

Registered nurses change locations and jobs about every two or three years, so they are exposed to a variety of working conditions during their time in the service. They might find themselves caring for the wounded in active war zones and might have reason to fear for their own safety and well-being. They might have to cope with stress from handling trauma cases, unremitting emergencies, and the tragic deaths of young people in their care. They might have to work with patients who carry infectious diseases such as COVID-19, taking precautions even as they have reasonable worries that they too could become sick.

Registered nurses assigned to work in military hospitals and clinics in the United States will have similar experiences as those in the civilian world, but there is always a chance that they will be deployed somewhere less hospitable. This was the case for Captain Dukes, who was deployed to Afghanistan. The weather there was often too hot, too cold, or too dry, and keeping anything clean was a constant challenge. And, certainly, Dukes faced danger when she was assigned to a war zone. She recalls,

> My team essentially worked out of a small plywood hospital. We were the first line of treatment for soldiers severely injured in combat. We had a small ER [emergency room], OR [operating room], and ICU [intensive care unit] typically staffing three nurses per section. We also had a few CRNA's [certified registered nurse anesthetists, who can safely sedate patients], general surgeons, Army medics, and other support staff. All in all, our medical unit had about 22 people. I was in charge of the emergency department which was essentially a two-bed trauma station. Patients would come in, be triaged [the process by which patients who are most ill are treated first] by the general surgeon, and either go directly to surgery or stay in the ER for an immediate intervention such as a chest tube [a thin tube for draining fluid from the lungs] if necessary.[18]

Opportunities for Advancement

As with other military jobs, RNs can expect automatic promotions in rank and increases in salary as they accumulate years of service. They enter the military as second lieutenants and can reach as high as a colonel in the Army.

Most RNs will start with duties centered on patient care. As their service continues, they may find themselves in supervisory positions. For example, they might become the head of nursing for an entire base. However, many RNs do not enter the profession to be leaders. One nurse who found a downside to moving away from patient care was Captain Dukes, who says,

> My only complaint about the Army Nurse Corps is that if you come in as a brand new nurse, by the time you hit the three-year mark the Army begins to want you to emphasize leadership over bedside nursing. You are put in a position of authority but still have relatively little clinical experience. You are still getting your bedside skills in check. I believe they are taking nurses away from patient care too early—people need time to become competent nurses. I was glad I entered the Army with some prior nursing experience.[19]

Employment Prospects
in the Civilian World

Registered nurses who are preparing to leave the armed forces can expect to have little difficulty finding jobs in the civilian world. Employment growth is expected to be 9 percent through 2030. Retirements and people leaving the profession are expected to add 175,900 jobs just by themselves. A large number of those jobs will be found in hospitals and outpatient care centers.

If they prefer, RNs can switch from active military duty to the reserves. That is what Harrie did when she left the Army. In the reserves, she works with logistics—helping to supervise the movement of troops and supplies to destinations around the world—as well as with medical units. She is convinced that being a military nurse has helped her to advance in her profession. "I left nursing school confident that I had a plan," she says. "I spent many years not only gaining clinical skills but having the ability to work independently in a respected profession. I was able to further my education with a master's in executive nursing and plan to get my MBA [master of business administration degree] as well. The Army was a great choice for me."[20]

What Does a Dental Assistant Do?

Dental assistants are invaluable members of dental practices, whether they are civilians or members of the military. As the name implies, they aid dentists, tackling administrative duties such as ordering supplies, scheduling appointments, keeping records, and making certain that dentists have all the sterilized tools they need for the procedures they are about to perform.

Dental assistants participate in procedures as well, passing tools to the dentist, holding the suction hose in the patient's mouth during dental procedures, and interacting with patients to make certain they are comfortable and aware of the importance of flossing and brushing. Some are trained to take and process dental X-rays. This career should not be confused with that of a dental hygienist, who specializes in cleaning teeth.

In the military, dental assistants are part of a team that ensures the health of personnel who may be deployed at a moment's notice. These military personnel cannot miss work because of poor dental health. "We want troops to be at their peak of health," says Angelica, who spent six years as a dental assistant in the Army before serving in the same capacity as

A Few Facts

Minimum Educational Requirements
High school diploma or equivalent

Personal Qualities
Dexterous, detail oriented, organized, good listener

Working Conditions
Dental offices and more remote locations

Salary
Varies by rank and years of service

Future Job Outlook
Steady hiring through next decade

a member of the Alaska National Guard and working for a civilian oral surgeon. "Being part of a team that helps serve our country's troops is amazing."[21]

Colonel James Kutner, a dental readiness consultant serving at Joint Base Langley-Eustis in Hampton, Virginia, notes that some service members in high-stress jobs are more likely to have dental issues than others. He explains,

> In theater [war zones and deployments], about 1-in-5 medical patients has a dental-related concern. We see acute gum disease, unanticipated eruption of third molars, fractured teeth from grinding and stress, and airmen with work-related oral injuries during their deployment. Having skilled dental teams in deployed areas ensures that we can return [military members] with dental emergencies to duty as soon as possible.[22]

A Typical Workday

Because members of the military are required to stay "in fighting shape," the typical day is likely to start very early in the morning with a workout. Some dental assistants might wake up early to get this training in before heading to the dental clinic or medical center to which they are assigned. Their days may begin with meetings in which the dental staff is apprised of what procedures are expected to be performed that day.

After the meetings, the dental assistants will make certain that everything is in place for the day's work, sterilizing tools, and stocking paper gowns and other often-used items. As patients arrive, the dental assistant will greet them, find out if there have been any changes in their health since their last visit, and take X-rays if they are due. Or, if a patient is there to have a cavity filled or similar procedure, the dental assistant will set everything up for the dentist and stand by to assist. The job generally has regular hours—such as 9 a.m. to 5 p.m. or 7 a.m. to 4 p.m.—and the dental assistant's day can be expected to go by quickly, with many patients coming and going.

Education and Training

Young people who want to start a health care career fairly quickly without needing a college degree may be drawn to dental assisting. Those who wish to join the military without having completed such training as a civilian will need to take the Armed Services Vocational Aptitude Battery (ASVAB). Free to take and available through some high schools, the ASVAB measures math, science, and communication and technology skills and is considered of average difficulty. The test determines aptitude for different types of careers offered by the military. To be assigned training as a dental assistant, however, applicants must earn a ninety-one or better out of ninety-nine points on the skilled technical portion of the test.

Before undergoing job training, applicants need to go through eight to ten weeks of basic combat training, depending on the branch of the service. Basic training is rigorous and includes classroom instruction, physical training, and instruction in weapons handling, survival skills, and military conduct.

Applicants who make it into the Air Force's dental assistant program spend forty-eight days at the branch's training school in Fort Hood, Texas, where their education includes classroom and lab work, hands-on and practical instruction, and an opportunity for supervised work with patients. The scenario is different for the Army, where dental assistant students receive thirty weeks of advanced individual training, which covers dental office procedures, oral hygiene techniques, and the skills required to take X-rays. Students study dental terminology, anatomy, microbiology, and physiology.

After graduating from tech school, dental assistants continue to learn on the job. Students can also study to be a certified dental assistant (CDA) through an exam given by the Dental Assisting National Board. The CDA is a national certification that can be earned while in the military or as a civilian.

Skills and Personality

Successful dental assistants share common traits. Individuals who are organized, have good dexterity, have a knack for following protocols or procedures, enjoy talking to people, and are capable of communicating well with dentists and their patients could be suited to this profession.

Dental assistants also have to be comfortable with putting their gloved fingers in a patient's mouth; being around blood, plaque (a sticky film on teeth and gums that can lead to decay and tooth loss), saliva, and needles; and taking orders from superiors. They have to learn aspects of anatomy and be equally at home learning in a classroom environment and on the job. Some are tasked with teaching less-experienced dental assistants how to do the job.

Working Conditions

Dental assistants usually work in well-appointed dental offices, but sometimes they work in temporary quarters under less-than-

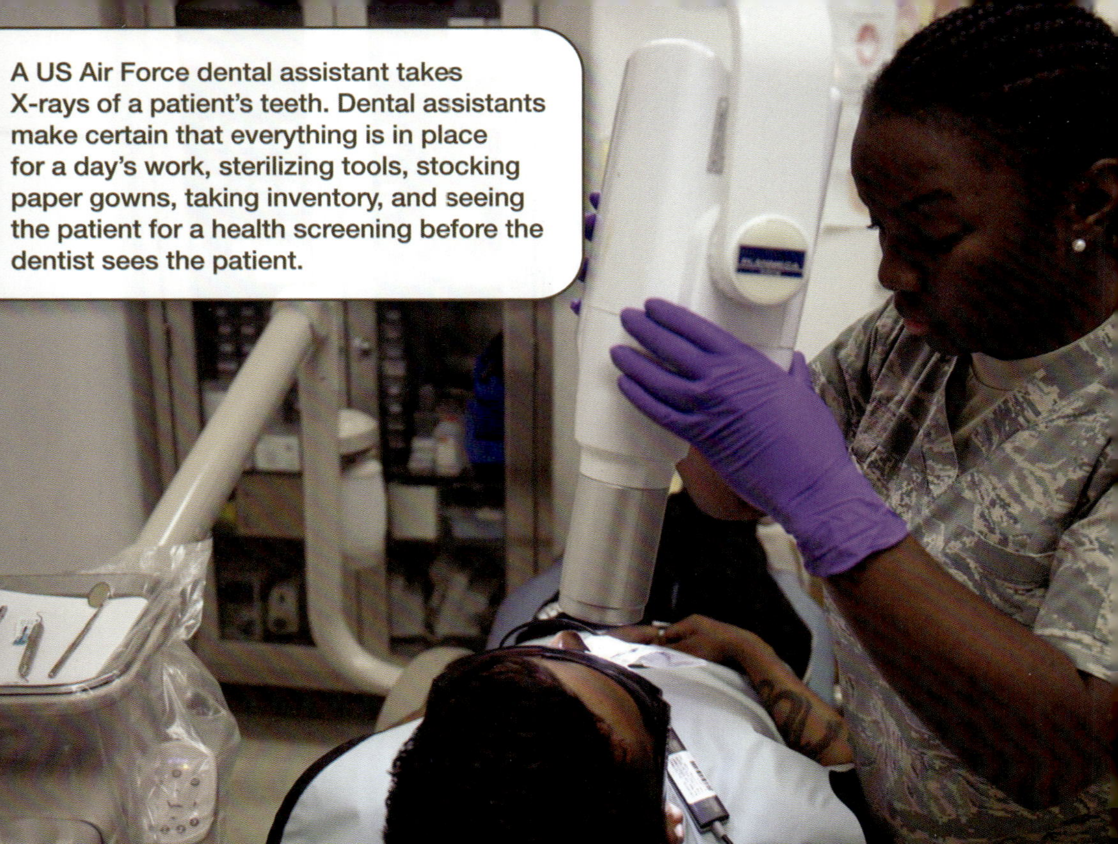

A US Air Force dental assistant takes X-rays of a patient's teeth. Dental assistants make certain that everything is in place for a day's work, sterilizing tools, stocking paper gowns, taking inventory, and seeing the patient for a health screening before the dentist sees the patient.

ideal conditions. The volume of work may be stressful at times, and the job requires standing throughout the day and bending over to work in the mouths of patients reclining in the examination rooms.

Writing on the job website Indeed, a former career dental assistant in the Army who had been stationed at Fort Jackson, South Carolina, comments,

The Army was a very disciplined and structured environment. It taught me how to talk to people and I got to meet people from different cultures and learn. I was able to learn how to properly work in a team. In order to do this, communication is the most important thing, instead of guessing [what] you and everyone has to do. The hardest part was trying to push yourself even if [you are] tired. But after a while it just becomes natural.[23]

Opportunities for Advancement

Dental assistants can rise in rank and increase their salaries as they accumulate more years of service. They can also continue their education while in the military, perhaps seeking out more training to become dental hygienists or even dentists. They may also have the opportunity to take leadership roles. Corporal Michelle Binder became a squad leader at Fort Bliss in Texas, where she was in charge of four soldiers and a training manager working with more than one hundred staffers at the dental care clinic. "Being a squad leader brings me the most joy," she comments. "I say this because I am learning and enjoying leading and guiding these soldiers. I know sometimes different situations are challenging, but it is also rewarding knowing that I can provide my guidance and advice for these soldiers."[24]

Employment Prospects in the Civilian World

With the employment of dental assistants projected to grow by 11 percent through 2029, transitioning into a civilian job should not be difficult. Some 23,400 new jobs are expected to be added in the field, according to the Bureau of Labor Statistics' *Occupational Outlook Handbook*. It represents a field poised for growth because of the surging numbers of older Americans. Older Americans will require more dental visits to fix or replace teeth that wear out, become diseased, or need other care. They are more likely to get gum disease and may need to visit their dental office every few months instead of every six months.

In the civilian world, dental assistants can choose to work in specialty dental practices, thus giving themselves the opportunity to work with different populations. For example, they might work with children (pediatric dentists), people with gum disease (periodontists), adolescents (orthodontists), or surgical patients (oral surgeons). And once trained as dental assistants, they may discover that they enjoy working in the dental area but would like more training, perhaps enrolling in a dental hygienist program.

Rebecca was a dental assistant in the Army who transitioned into a similar civilian role. She says, "Working for the US Army was a great experience for me. I am very grateful for my time with the Army because it gave me a sense of satisfaction that I could give back to those who serve. I wanted to give all our soldier patients the care and professionalism that I would want for my family members. I met many people from all over the United States and foreign countries, made a lot of friends and got to work with some great patients."[25]

What Does a Physical Therapist Do?

Whether they sit at a desk all day or are headed to the battlefield, soldiers and sailors need to be ready to do their jobs. Physical therapists (PTs) work with the body's nerves, muscles, joints, and bones to prevent injuries, minimize their impact, and help people regain functions after the injuries occur. Military members with desk jobs may suffer from back pain because of poor posture or may experience pain from repetitive motion, such as striking a keyboard all day. Military personnel with more active jobs may develop pain from, for example, carrying 140 pounds of equipment, such as weapons and backpacks filled with ammunition, water, batteries, and food. PTs are also called on to help people who are injured in combat, including those who lose limbs and may need to adjust to life in a wheelchair or with an artificial limb. They also work with people who suffer strokes or paralysis or need to recover from knee replacements and other surgeries.

When a service member complains of muscle pain or weakness or has difficultly walking or running, for example, he or she may be referred to a PT to determine why and to receive an individualized therapy plan. Physical therapists in the Army, Navy, or Air Force order

A Few Facts

Minimum Educational Requirements
Doctorate degree in physical therapy

Personal Qualities
Decisive, dexterous, analytical, and even tempered

Working Conditions
Hospitals, clinics, field units

Salary
Varies by rank and length of service

Future Job Outlook
Ongoing high demand

imaging studies to find the cause. Imaging technologies, such as magnetic resonance imaging, computerized tomography scans, and X-rays, allow medical professionals to "see" inside the body from the outside.

Physical therapists also evaluate soldiers' readiness for combat. Active-duty members of the military have to pass periodic fitness tests. PTs not only administer the tests but also work with individuals who have difficulty passing them. They work with these individuals to build up their stamina and help them practice the exercises that they find difficult.

Variety is built into the physical therapist's job. They oversee the work of therapy technicians, who order supplies, clean equipment, take notes on patient progress, and assist with some movement activities. PTs also confer with surgeons and other medical doctors caring for their patients. They may be part of a team that includes strength and conditioning coaches and exercise physiologists— medical experts who tell patients how to improve their health through exercise plans created specifically for them. They also work with social workers whose role is to see that patients have all the services they need to recover from their injuries. Social workers may refer patients to PTs, and PTs may refer patients to social workers.

Lieutenant Erin Kocher has been working with sailors for nearly five years at Naval Hospital Twentynine Palms in California. She says, "I really love the aspect of working one-on-one with a patient. Getting them back to doing something that they love, whether it's working out, playing sports, or just being able to play with their children again without pain is hugely rewarding."[26]

A Typical Workday

On a typical workday, Jeff Turner, an Air Force PT and deputy flight commander of physical therapy at Peterson Air Force Base in Colorado Springs, Colorado, sees about a dozen patients. But he has been busy even before he sees his first patients at around 9:30 a.m. His day starts with about forty-five minutes of working on his own body through flight physical training, weight lifting, or playing a group sport. He arrives at the base clinic to spend nearly two hours meeting with associates, including the technicians whom he supervises. During this time, he looks over image studies he ordered and acquaints himself with new patient referrals ordered by other doctors. Only then does he see his first patients that day, usually six of them in three hours.

His lunch break lasts an hour, but he often uses part of that time to meet with team members and enter notes he made for the patients he has just seen. His afternoon is spent seeing an additional six patients for three hours before meeting with his colleagues again, working on his notes, and leaving for home at about 4:30 p.m. According to Turner,

> Military physical therapy demands simple, effective, and efficient medical care at a minimum. My evaluation emphasizes ruling out sinister stuff, reassuring and educating, and promoting self-care and independence. A visit with me usually consists of 60 percent education/advice/reassurance/strategic health planning, 30 percent exercise demonstration/prescription, and 10 percent manual therapy.[27]

Education and Training

Military PTs must have a doctorate in the discipline from an accredited university or attend the military's own school located at Fort Sam Houston in San Antonio, Texas. Students admitted to the Texas program do not pay tuition and receive a salary and financial assistance toward their housing and living expenses while in school. This is a big plus for many students. According to a 2020 report from the American Physical Therapy Association, the average physical therapy program graduate accumulates more than $116,000 in tuition debt. Students who attend nonmilitary PT training programs before joining the military are eligible to receive government assistance in paying off their college loans.

Students can apply to PT programs after they have a bachelor of science degree and a solid grounding in anatomy, chemistry, social sciences, and physics. They also need a high grade point average and a high score on the Graduate Record Exam, a test students must take to be accepted to graduate school. Students typically earn their doctorates in three years. Those who join the military as they train agree to serve for seven and a half years: three or four as active members and the remainder in the reserves.

During physical therapy school, they will spend time in a classroom, laboratory, and, eventually, working with patients under supervision. They will study anatomy; cellular histology (the study of cells under a microscope); physiology; exercise physiology; kinesiology and biomechanics (related studies of the way bodies move); neuroscience; pharmacology; behavioral sciences; ethics; and heart, lung, hormone, metabolic, and musculoskeletal systems. After completing their education, they must pass the National Physical Therapy Examination given by the Federation of State Boards of Physical Therapy. Passing this exam leads to a license to practice. PTs who want to specialize undergo additional education in their chosen areas.

Skills and Personality

Young people thinking about training as physical therapists may want to inventory their personality and skill set. Do they have a desire to help people? Will they be comfortable working with amputees and people in pain? Are they good at communicating information? Would they enjoy manipulating their patients' limbs or demonstrating exercises and proper form that will help individuals achieve results?

There are other qualities that are important to possess or nurture too. Physical therapists need good time-management skills so they can juggle many different duties and cases and referrals in a single eight-hour day. They need to have good hand-eye coordination and problem-solving abilities. Moreover, as members of the military, they also have to be willing to follow established protocols and to respect people who have higher ranks than they do. And because they work with people's bodies, they need to understand how muscles and joints work and what happens when disease or injuries impact their functioning. These professionals need to know what is possible as people recover from their impairments and to make the best possible use of the tools available to them: walkers, canes, wheelchairs, balance balls, treadmills, resistance bands, injections, and medications.

Working Conditions

Military PTs work in hospitals and in clinics on military bases. They sometimes work in temporary or mobile units that are located in areas of the greatest need, such as near war zones or where catastrophes are taking place and humanitarian missions are present. When they are working near a combat zone or as part of a humanitarian mission, military PTs will be working in temporary

Creating Better Runners

It may seem as though anyone can run well with no instruction, but Captain Anthony Williams, a PT in the Army, knows that is not true. As part of his duties, Williams has taught running workshops at Camp Buehring in the Middle Eastern nation of Kuwait. Williams points out that soldiers often have to run in the course of their duties, so PTs are often called on to help them reduce the risk of running-related injuries.

Soldiers tend to strike the ground with their heels when they run, Williams says, but they would suffer fewer injuries if they strike it with the middle of their foot. "When we decrease the length of our stride and increase the number of steps we take, we reduce the impact on our joints," he explains.

One soldier who benefited from the training is Private Michael Radice. "I learned that I'm a novice runner even though I've been in the Army for a year now," he says. "I thought I knew how to run, just like anyone else in the Army, but Captain Williams was able to show me some of my issues."

Quoted in Liane Hatch, "U.S. Army Physical Therapist Teaches Running Technique to Kuwait National Guard," U.S. Army Central, April 30, 2019. www.usarcent.army.mil.

structures where there is less equipment and where amenities such as heat, air-conditioning, and good lighting may be absent.

Opportunities for Advancement

Physical therapists enter the military as officers and leaders, with the rank of captain or lieutenant, depending on the service branch. They can expect to achieve higher ranks and pay increases the longer they are in the service. They will also be reassigned multiple times and may end up running clinics and being given greater responsibilities. Physical therapists can also opt to continue their education by specializing in orthopedics (working with injured bones and muscles) or geriatrics (working with elderly patients). They can apply for residencies and fellowships in those areas. As Major Eric Walter, a PT with the Air Force, explains,

There are multiple career paths that the Air Force can guide you into such as research, leadership, or [being] embedded into units. You can sign up for jobs outside of our career field to get a better scope of the military life. You are the limiting factor of what you can imagine you could do with a career in the Air Force. If you are bored as an Air Force PT, that's likely your own doing.[28]

Employment Prospects in the Civilian World

When it comes time to leave the military, PTs should have few difficulties finding jobs in the civilian sector. Job growth in this field is well above average at 22 percent, with forty-nine thousand new positions expected to be added through 2030. The growth is being driven by an aging population and health insurance companies—which pay for a large percentage of the cost of treating injured patients—that want to keep injuries from leading to debilitation and additional health concerns. Those returning to the civilian world may find jobs in hospitals, private practices, nursing homes, and patients' homes.

Introduction: An Essential Role

1. Quoted in Jennifer Garvin, "Life in the Air Force Dental Corps," *ADA News*, September 18, 2018. www.ada.org.

Physician

2. Quoted in 81st Medical Group, "National Doctors' Day: Being a Medical Doctor in the Air Force," Keesler Air Force Base, March 30, 2018. www.keesler.af.mil.
3. Quoted in Julia Birkinbine Poulter, "A Military Doctor Talks Deployments, Maternity Leave, and the Challenges She Faces as an Army Mom," *The Everymom*, November 11, 2020. https://theeverymom.com.
4. Quoted in Rose Raymond, "The Navy Paid for This Doctor's Medical Education. Here's How He Fared," *The DO*, May 17, 2017. https://thedo.osteopathic.org.
5. Kevin Jubbal, "So You Want to Be a Military Doctor," Med School Insiders, February 22, 2020. https://medschoolinsiders.com.
6. Quoted in Brendan Murphy, "Are Medical School Service Scholarships Right for You?," American Medical Association, October 16, 2019. www.ama-assn.org.

Pharmacist

7. Quoted in Jane Lee, "BMACH Pharmacy: Like Mother, like Daughter," US Army, September 14, 2021. www.army.mil.
8. Quoted in Lee, "BMACH Pharmacy."
9. Erin Mays, "Reality Versus Expectation: The First Year of Pharmacy School," IDstewardship.com, October 19, 2017. www.idstewardship.com.
10. Quoted in Jordan Kellerman, "For Two Graduates, Balancing School and the Military Became Second Nature," Skaggs School of Pharmacy and Pharmaceutical Sciences, May 18, 2021. https://news.cuanschutz.edu.
11. Quoted in Ryan Marotta, "The Call to Military Service," *Pharmacy Times*, August 4, 2015. www.pharmacytimes.com.
12. Quoted in Kate Traynor, "Resilience Critical for Army Pharmacists," American Society of Health-System Pharmacists, May 1, 2019. www.ashp.org.

Laboratory Specialist

13. Quoted in Russell Toof, "On the Frontlines Against COVID: Medical Laboratory Specialist," US Army, June 10, 2020. www.army.mil.
14. Quoted in Medical Laboratory Observer, "Where the Heroes Are: A Tribute to Military MLTs," December 1, 2003. www.mlo-online.com.
15. Quoted in Douglas Stutz, "I Am Navy Medicine—and Laboratory Technician—HM1 KC Geisler," Defense Visual Information Distribution Service, April 21, 2021. www.dvidshub.net.
16. Quoted in Medical Laboratory Observer, "Where the Heroes Are."

Registered Nurse

17. Quoted in ThriveAP, "An Inside Look into Life as an Army Nurse," *Nurse Practitioner Career Advice* (blog), October 23, 2018. https:// thriveap.com.
18. Quoted in ThriveAP, "An Inside Look into Life as an Army Nurse."
19. Quoted in ThriveAP, "An Inside Look into Life as an Army Nurse."
20. Quoted in RegisteredNursing.org, "Guide to Military Nursing Education & Service: True Stories from the Field, Army Nurse Corps," July 28, 2021. www.registerednursing.org.

Dental Assistant

21. Quoted in Dental Assistant Life, "Why These Dental Assistants Love Their Military Careers," July 2, 2019. www.dentalassistantlife.org.
22. Quoted in Peter Holstein, "Say 'Aaaaaah'—Air Force Deployed Dental Teams Support Readiness," Air Force Medical Service, October 20, 2017. www.airforcemedicine.af.mil.
23. Quoted in Indeed, comment on "U.S. Army Employee Reviews for Dental Assistant," April 15, 2019. https://indeed.com.
24. Quoted in Melissa Tennen, "Serving Those Who Serve: Dental Assistants Forge Military Careers," *Inside Dental Assisting*, May/June 2013, vol. 9, no. 3. www.aegisdentalnetwork.com.
25. Quoted in Dental Assistant Life, "Why These Dental Assistants Love Their Military Careers."

Physical Therapist

26. Quoted in David Marks, "Navy Physical Therapist Embodies the Four P's: People, Platforms, Performance and Power," Defense Virtual Information Distribution Service, December 21, 2020. www .dvidshub.net.
27. Quoted in Jeffrey Turner, "Spotlight: An Interview with Military PT, Jeff Turner, PT, DPT," *CoreCentral* (blog), Core Medical Group, 2021. https://blog.coremedicalgroup.com.
28. Eric Walter, "You Can Be a Military PT," *The Pulse* (blog), American Physical Therapy Association, April 28, 2020. www.ptcas.org.

Scott Snyder is an active-duty Navy physician. He has served in the Navy for eight years. He joined the Navy while still in medical school. Snyder spoke about his career by telephone.

Q: Why did you join the Navy?

A: I joined the Navy to serve my country and be a part of something bigger than myself. My mom was in the Army National Guard as a nurse before I was born, and my grandfather was in the Army and served in World War II. That exposure inspired me. I specifically joined the Navy because I like the ocean and being on the water. I figured that would allow me to match my desire to be near the water and serve the country.

Q: Why did you become a physician?

A: My mom was a nurse, so I got to see a little bit of the hospital when I was younger. We had a close family friend who was a physician, and I got to observe him during high school and was able to see what he did. And that exposure let me become a physician. I was an emergency medical technician in high school and college, so I got to see what prehospital medical care looked like and was able to serve my local community; all of that contributed to my desire to become a physician. Even as a little child I knew I wanted to be a doctor, and that was the path I took in high school in the courses I took. Some of the courses that were helpful were biology, chemistry, and anatomy. I was able to take Advanced Placement Biology as a junior and an anatomy elective as a high school senior.

Q: How did you train for this career?

A: It started in high school with taking challenging courses, with really pushing myself and getting good grades as well as doing extracurricular activities that made me well-rounded. In college, I studied chemistry and biology and was in a premedical focus. Medical school is four years; it gives you the basic knowledge and training on how to be a physician. In your third and fourth years in medical school, you do rotations in various specialties and then you pick the one you like most. I chose internal medicine, which is focused on hospital-based care and complex care for adults. The internal medicine residency was three years with a combination of hospital-based and clinic-based rotations. After medical school residency, I chose to do a two-year fellowship in geriatric and palliative care, which is focused on older and frailer adults with complex medical issues. All in all, total training was thirteen years.

Q: How would you describe your typical workday?

A: I'm a primary care doctor in a clinic on a military base, so my day at work starts at 7:30 and we have a morning clinic meeting to talk about the day and then we start seeing patients at 8 a.m. Most visits are twenty minutes, with a maximum of twenty patients per day. We have a short lunch break and then see patients until 4 p.m. These are a mix of in-person visits and telemedicine visits where I am talking to people on the phone.

Q: How stressful is your job?

A: Many of the days are stressful because we have to make a lot of decisions in a short amount of time, given the number of patients we see. Each decision has many aspects to consider.

Q: What do you like most about your job?

A: Dealing with the patients. As a doctor, that's what we are trained to do. I really enjoy interacting with them and helping them improve their health.

Q: What do you like least about your job?
A: As a Navy clinic doctor, the demands are similar to a civilian clinic doctor. What I like least about my job is the small amount of time we get to spend with patients. Having to complete a lot of paperwork means spending less time with patients. In the last two years, I have seen an increase in paperwork requirements.

Q: What personal qualities do you find most valuable for this type of work?
A: Flexibility with what the day throws at you is important. There's a lot of pressure to perform at the highest level because people are relying on your decisions and your critical thinking. Honesty and integrity are also important, to always do what is right for the patient and especially now in the age of misinformation, holding true to that is important. Even if someone is disagreeing with you, standing firm in your evidence-based knowledge is important.

Q: What advice do you have for students who might be interested in a career as a military physician?
A: There are multiple branches of the military that a physician could join: the Army, Navy, Air Force, and—less well-known— the US Public Health Service. So, if someone is interested in joining the military, they should look at them all and choose the one that makes the most sense for them. No matter what job you take in the military, it has unique burdens given the type of service required.

Other Medical Careers in the Military

Animal care specialist
Audiologist
Biomedical specialist
Clinical laboratory scientist
Dental hygienist
Dentist
Dermatologist
Hospital corpsman
Industrial hygiene officer
Infectious disease officer
Medevac medic
Microbiologist
Neurologist
Nuclear medicine officer
Nurse practitioner
Obstetrician

Occupational therapist
Operating room specialist
Optician
Optometrist
Palliative care doctor
Pediatrician
Pharmacy tech
Physician assistant
Practical nurse
Preventative medicine
  specialist
Psychologist
Registered dietician
Trauma surgeon
Urologist
Veterinarian

Editor's note: The online *Occupational Outlook Handbook* of the US Department of Labor's Bureau of Labor Statistics is an excellent source of information on jobs in hundreds of career fields, including many of those listed here. The *Occupational Outlook Handbook* may be accessed online at www.bls.gov/ooh.

Bureau of Labor Statistics

www.bls.gov/ooh/military/military-careers.htm

This government website includes the *Occupational Outlook Handbook*, which offers extensive information on military careers, including what their duties are, how to train for them, and what they pay, as well as careers that are considered similar.

Commissioned Corps of the US Public Health Service

www.usphs.gov

This is the official website of the US Public Health Service, a service branch devoted to public health that employs six thousand officers, including physicians, nurses, dentists, dieticians, and veterinarians, at eight hundred locations around the world. The website provides information on possible careers, the service's history, and the places where people work.

Military.com

www.military.com

This website provides news on what is happening in the military and resources for veterans and their families. It includes information on military life, joining the service, and military history.

Operation Military Kids

www.operationmilitarykids.org

The website is designed for young people who are interested in the military. All entries are written by veterans and cover such topics as how to choose a branch of service, what to ask a recruiter, and understanding the military alphabet.

Today's Military

www.todaysmilitary.com

This US Department of Defense website offers an excellent overview of career options, career stories, benefits, schooling, and more. Visitors to the website can learn about boot camp, becoming an officer, and the Armed Services Vocational Aptitude Battery.

US Air Force

www.airforce.com

This is the official website of the Air Force. The careers section provides information on a variety of careers and is organized by areas of interest.

US Army

www.goarmy.com

This official website lets visitors explore career options in the Army. Visitors can take a quiz to see what careers their interests might suggest, learn how to join the Army, get details about basic training, and see how to find the Army on Facebook, Twitter, Instagram, and more.

US Coast Guard

www.gocoastguard.com

The Coast Guard's official website offers information about active-duty and reserve careers. Visitors can explore active-duty and reserve options, ask questions, and connect with the Coast Guard through social media.

US Navy

www.navy.com

Visitors to this website can explore all the career options available through the Navy based on individual aspirations and interests. Brochures can be downloaded that explain how to join, the benefits of doing so, officer programs, and more.

Index

Picture Credits

Cover: Gardinovachki/Shutterstock.com

6: Maury Aaseng
12: Mass Communication Specialist 2nd Class Eric C. Tretter/United States Navy
26: Mass Communication Specialist 3rd Class Jake Greenberg/United States Navy
34: dpa picture alliance/Alamy Stock Photo
42: Ted Small/Alamy Stock Photo

About the Author

Gail Snyder is a freelance writer and advertising copywriter who has written more than twenty-five books for young readers. She has a degree in journalism from Pennsylvania State University and lives in Chalfont, Pennsylvania, with her husband, Hal Marcovitz.